You're Not Your Boobs!

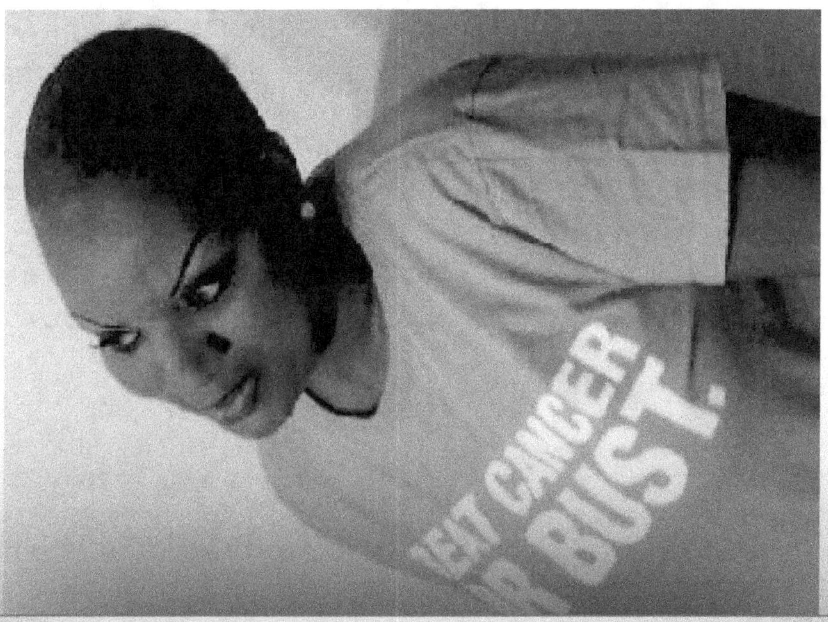

by Teresa Graham

For it is God which worketh in you both to will and to do of his good pleasure (Philippians 2:13).

Be Advised: Horrific Photos Have Been Included Within This Book. You Will See Pictures Of The Cancer Eating My Flesh, Please Keep Photos Away From Your Children!

You're Not Your Boobs

A True Story

"For I will restore health unto thee, and I will heal thee of thy wounds, saith the LORD; (Jeremiah 30:17).

....

....

....

....

"O LORD my God, I cried to You for help, and You healed me" (Psalm 30:2).

"Pull me out of the net that they have laid privily for me: for thou art my strength" (Psalm 31:4).

Presented To ________________________

BY ________________________

Special Occasion ________________________

____

Date ________________________

Put The Gloves Up! You Already Won!

You're Not Your Boobs

A True Story

ISBN: 13:978-19758884345

ISBN: 10-1975884345

Printed in the United States of America.

DEDICATION

This book is dedicated to my friend, Irene Havy, you left this life too soon, you were so precious and you are irreplaceable! I will always love you more than words can say. With my tears, I would say, I was proud to be your friend. But someday, I have the faith to know we will see each other again! Rest on my sister until we meet again.

My sister Marietta I. McTaw, thanks for the title of this book, it has served the writing in this book very well.

This book is also dedicated to my doctors and to women from around the world who have battled this deadly diseased called cancer: I pray that this book will be a vital part of healing and will restore your hearts as you read through the pages of this book. ————Dr. Teresa Graham

Contents

"For I will restore health unto thee, and I will heal thee of thy wounds, saith the Lord;" (Jeremiah 30:17).

INTRODUCTION

Cancer was lurking around in the darkest parts of my body. Waiting to introduce itself to the surface of my flesh, battling viciously against my healthy cells, for its right to squeeze the life from my body. The shadow of its stronghold follows closely, as it recruit other cancer cells to join in with them to stage my early demise. It filled my breast with the disease of death, seeking to melt away my health.

Battling Viciously Against My Healthy Cells

It came like a thief in the night, laying dormant in the shadows of my body, transforming my physical appearance into an unknown stranger, looking back at my reflection in the mirror, hearing voices of fear in my mind screaming, "Soon your flesh will be laying in a grave with worms covering every inch of your body."

As I stood silently crying for five minutes gazing into the mirror at the new me, the unrecognizable person brought tears to my eyes wishing this nightmare would be over soon.

There were so many puzzling questions as to why God would allowed this happen to His prophet. I had become so frustrated until it had become unnerving to me. Its like I went to bed one night and woke up with a tree sticking out of my side, it just doesn't make any sense.

As I leaned against the mirror to take a closer look the scars on my chest, the thought of having my boobs back was beating me like a drummer beats his drums. My mind was definitely running out of control. The cancer didn't have any regards for the life I lived before it decided to show up throwing a monkey wrench in my ministry. It was there to shake my faith in God, and eat my flesh like a raven lion rips apart its prey.

Introduction

I was left to make the decision to have the nine hour surgery to stop this deadly aggressive cancer from spreading and causing my demise.

You're Not Your Boobs was written as a motivational book and as therapy for me too accept my new fake boobs. The title came through a conversation my sister Marietta, and I shared over the phone. I had made a statement about my breast and she said,

"You're Not Your Boobs!" Immediately after she made that statement, a light bulb went off, and here you have this awesome book in the palm of your hands as a good read today!

It is my prayers that you read it and apply Scripture as you walk through the window of my eyes. This book is my heartfelt testimony of a wrestle within the attic of my mind, and how God was there through the **surgeries, chemotherapy, radiations, test** and **scans.** In know way was this book written to replace your doctors medical advice.

In this book I wish to publicly thank all of the ***doctors, nurses, medical staffs, family*** and ***friends*** who daily prayed for me, and showed love through their flowers, cards and phone calls.

Most importantly, I thank ***God-Jehovah-Rapha*** for healing my body through ***Jesus Christ's*** sacrifice on the cross.

"Surely he hath borne our griefs, and carried our sorrows: yet we did esteem him stricken, smitten of God, and afflicted. But he was wounded for our transgressions, he was bruised for our iniquities: the chastisement of our peace was upon him; and with his stripes we are healed" (Isaiah 53:4-5).

He Hath Borne Our Griefs,

CHAPTER ONE

Where Do I Begin?

The beginning of this book was birth seven years ago in North

Carolina's hospice center. Irene had been fighting stomach cancer for

five months, and she was getting weaker by the moment.

Five months before her diagnosis Irene complains of always

having to burp and pass gas. She thought it was something she had

eaten, but asked me what I thought it could be. I implored her to get

her blood check. She just brush me off for months, holding onto her

beliefs she was fine. I had pushed hard for Irene to get a check up

from her doctor. Then came the decision to call the doctor for an

appointment.

The day I received her phone call, was one of the most devastating days of my life. I was having a great day. I have just started my television ministry on the community cable channel. Then all of a sudden the phone rings and I grab it, "Hi Teresa, I'm going to the doctor in the next hour, will you pray for me?" She asked. I stood smiling with my hands raised in praise, "Yes, do you want to party now?"

"Not now Teresa, but when you do pray, please ask God what's the reason behind my burping, I know God will give you the answer, and when I return home, I will call for my answer" she said.

I stood still, stun by her statement still stun by her statement. A huge smiles spread across my face.

"What makes you think that?" I asked.

"You've spoken things in my life that was true. God is the only one who could've reveal those secrets to you."

I had position my hand on my face as I started laughing, "Well, I take no glory, all glory belongs to the father, let's wait and see what he has to say about your doctors appointment" I said jokingly.

"I can't wait to hear all about it" she said before hanging up the phone.

I stood and walked over to the kitchen sink staring out the window at the birds sitting on the fence. The early rays of the sun Shining through the window as I quietly talk to the Lord.

Quietly I asked, "Lord, my friend says she is going to see the doctor today! What's wrong with her?" I asked.

Typically, it would take 2 to 3 days before my answer would come from a prayer. Suddenly as I stood staring out the window for a few seconds the voice of the Lord said in a firm calm Voice, "She has cancer, and she is going to die."

Immediately I swallowed and to a deep breath. In a quick second, I was shocked and bewildered. Now desperately wanting to avoid talking with Irene, after hearing from God, I decided to avoid Irene's call, I needed to get my thoughts together before talking to her. I have to admit I didn't want to reveal or confirm what I knew would be her destiny.

The first sound I heard when I woke up with the phone ringing in my ears. I took a quick glance at the clock before answering the phone.

"Good morning Irene, how are you doing?" I asked.

"Hi Teresa, I called you on yesterday to hear what God revealed to you" she said.

Listen to herself voice, I sense she had been given bad news to confirm what God has revealed to me through prayer. Slowly, I set straight up in my bed, looking up at the ceiling, trying to fight back my emotions, hesitated to reveal what God has revealed to me. My eyes filled with tears as I revealed these life-changing words to my best friend.

"Irene, girl, please tell me what the doctor said," I shouted.

Irene started laughing, "No Teresa, you tell me what God has told you," she said.

I covered the phone with my hand and took a deep breath, wiping my eyes as the tears roll down my cheek saying quietly, oh lord! This is a bad day for me to be your prophet.

"Irene, the Lord said, you have cancer," I said with such sympathy.

"Well, Teresa, you definitely heard from God," she muttered, during my visit with the doctor, he has discovered I have stomach cancer, and I was given six months to live. But, I believe God will heal me, and I'm going to be fine, right Teresa?" She asked.

I fought back the flowing tears that washed my cheeks, placing my hands over the phone, trying to muffle the display of my pain. I gathered my courage to quote Isaiah 53:4-5 where it says, "Surely our griefs He himself bore, And our sorrows He carried: Yet we ourselves esteemed Him stricken, Smitten of God, and afflicted. But He was pierced through for our transgressions. He was crushed for our iniquities; The chastening for our well-being fell upon Him And by his scourging we are healed."

I had to quote "that scripture to get her to examine her thoughts, her healing, and her confession."

As I sit with the phone held up against my ear, I could hear in soft voice the denial and hurt, and a determination to prove the doctor's diagnosis was a flat out lie. The only thing I could say at that time was "If its God's will, you will be healed" I said.

Irene continued to speak with great faith and with enthusiasm as she made her faith known. REALITY was spoken by God on the day before. I didn't know rather to "cry or run, and as shocking as the news was, she really believed in her heart that God was going to heal her from cancer. I was still stun by the news god gave me yesterday in prayer, and here she was carrying on a bout her healing."

She has cancer and she is going to die

It is seem like her faith in God has grown a lot since we first met years ago, in the Christian bookstore, I owned and operated.

Where Do I Begin

She had been working as a sales person for this and company, seven asked to businesses. At first meeting, she had appear to be quite witty.

Perhaps, Irene was a little too witty.

She has a business and beauty radiating from her being. She was a woman about her business, and she was out to pitch her sale to me. As I stood is listening to her, I heard the Holy Ghost say, "She's not saved."

I continued to listen without saying a word, immediately after her long sales pitch, I grabbed her hand and said, "Do you know Jesus?"

She stood in shock as she looked at me with a look of surprise and humility. She started crying as she lowered her head and wiped her eyes. She said softly, I don't know Jesus, who is He?" she asked.

I immediately grabbed her hand, and rushed her through the store into my Office. I politely ask her to have a seat, let's talk.

She was about to meet Jesus Christ in the store!

I looked Irene in her eyes and begin to expose things that was going on in her household as the Holy Spirit revealed them to me.

Her mouth open wide, as she sat listening with a surprising look upon her face. As to say, "Who is this woman telling me all about myself?"

Remember when Jesus told the woman at the well all about herself. The Bible says, *"There cometh a woman of Samar'-ri-a to draw water: Jesus saith unto her, Give me to drink. (For his disciples were gone away unto the city to buy meat). Then saith the woman of Samari-a unto him, How is it that thou, being a Jew, askest drink of me, which am a woman of Sa-ma'ri-a? For the Jews have no dealings with the Sa-mar'ri-tans. Jesus answered and said unto her, If thou knewest the gift of God, and who it is that saith to thee, Give me to drink; thou wouldest have asked of him, and he would have given thee living water. The woman saith unto him, Sir, thou hast nothing to draw with, and the well is deep: from whence then hast thou that living water? Art thou greater than our father Jacob, which gave us the well, and drank thereof himself, and his children, and his cattle?*

Jesus answered and said unto her, whosoever drinketh of this water shall thirst again: But whosoever drinketh of the water that I shall give him shall never thirst; but the water that I shall give him shall be in him a well of water springing up into everlasting life.

The woman saith unto him, Sir, give me this water, that I thirst not, neither come hither to draw. Jesus saith unto her, Go call thy husband, and come hither. The woman answered and said, I have no husband. Jesus said unto her; Thou hast well said, I have no husband: For thou hast had five husbands: and he whom thou hast is not thy husband: in that saidst thou truly. The woman saith unto him, Sir, I perceive that thou art a prophet" (John 4:7-19).

Irene rubbed her temple and ask, "Teresa, are you saying you're a prophet" she asked.

I sat rubbing my hands together with a slight smile, "Yes," I said.

"How do you become a prophet, and what does a prophet do?"

There's Prophets Still On The Land Today!

"According to the Book of 2 Chronicles 24:19——God sent his prophets among them to leave them back to them. The Lord spoke to Jeremiah calling him his prophet. A prophets job is to **"pull down, destroy, root out, throw down, build** and **plant,** and to be the **mouth for God."** A prophet is born and chosen by God, not made by man. Irene, I was born in a prophet, and God confirmed it through the Bible."

"How did you confirm it, and what was His exact words?" she asked. I lean back in my chair and crossed my legs in order to get her attention making eye contact with her as I begin sharing my call from God as His prophet.

"One day, I was sitting on my school bus reading the Bible, asking God to confirm the office he hand-picked and anointed to me for. He said, turn to Jeremiah 1:1-10 revealing through Scripture my office, and after I read the Scriptures out loud, I heard his voice say, this is whom I called you to be a prophet to the nations."

"Wow Teresa," she said. Immediately after revealing my office

Where Do I Begin

from Ephesians 4:11-13 where it says, and he gave some, apostles; and some, prophets; and some, evangelists; and some, pastors and teachers; for the perfecting of the saints, for the work of the ministry, for the edifying of the body of Christ: within seconds Irene gave her life to the Lord, she had received salvation by confessing with her mouth the Lord Jesus and believing in her heart that God has raised Him from the dead and because of her confession she was saved and the angels was rejoicing in heaven over her.

That was the very first day, she had become a new person and the old life gone; a new life has begun.

My experience with the prophetic has been an awesome journey. I would only speak what I hear the Lord say, and nothing more, because a hold office sacred. Secondly, I never want to be out of the will of the father, and spoken of as a lying prophet.

After a few months had passed by, Irene, call crying hysterical.

"Teresa, I'm getting weaker, and when I look in the mirror I've seen nothing but a skeleton looking back at me," she said.

"Teresa, God isn't listening to me, I can't eat, and I'm having pain when I lay down, and I'm losing weight, Teresa. Please tell me what all did God tell you?" She asked.

I sat on the bed crossing my legs, preparing to speak with the voice of God has spoken concerning her life. I could tell by the tone of Irene voice she wanted me to reassure God's healing power would heal her body. Calmly I responded, "Irene, here is what the Lord said during my prayer. He said, "She has cancer and she is going to die!" I could tell the new shot heard to the core because she became silent over the phone. Then, within seconds, I could hear her soft sobs.

Over the next few months, I'd been praying for God to change his mind and add more years to her life. I had become desperate to a point, I started bargaining with God. Only to hear him say, "I have spoken." Each morning, I work up with the hope of God changing his mind. At the same time, fasting and praying for her life. The following morning, Irene called with a disturbing dream. "Teresa, she said, I had a dream of beautiful green grass on this strange land, and there was this strange man dancing in circles with me in his arms, and then I saw this a white blanket draped over the back of the bench," she said.

Immediately after hearing her dream, I knew her time heck come for her to leave us and go home to God. At that point, I started encouraging her to go to join her mother who lived in North Carolina. I felt at that time she really needed to spend Quality time loving on her family, comforting them and making sure they understood she will be okay.

When the Time change for her to die, she was surrounded by her loving family, who loved her more than life. We stood around her bed with him book in hand, sending spiritual hymns as we watch her slowly——very slowly.

What a memorable moment we'd experienced. This is unexpected defeat Hurt me. I felt trapped in my emotions, mad with God for not healing my friend.   24.

I don't claim to understand God's reason for Irène death, I'm convinced her death was in His perfect plan. Some people are convinced that death is a bad thing, when their loved one die, they lose their mind and make haste decisions without seeking God.

Apostle Paul, is considered one of the most important figures of the Apostolic age in the mid-30s-50s AD, he wrote about when a person dies they are present with the Lord.

Paul says, *"For we know that if our earthly House oh this tabernacle were dissolved, we have a building oh God, a house not made with hands, eternal in the heaven: is so be that being clothed we shall not be found naked. For we that are in this tabernacle do groan, being burdened: not for that we would be unclothed, but clothed upon, that mortality might be swallowed up of life. Now he that hath wrought us for the selfsame thing is God, who also hath given unto us the earnest of the Spirit. Therefore we are always confident, knowing that, whilst we are at home in the body, we are absent from the Lord;"*

(2 Corinthians 5:1-6).

Where Do I Begin

If you examine the Scriptures, you will find that Paul is revealing it's a good thing to die. The truth is that everyone wants to get to heaven, but nobody wants to die.

I can't speak or think for people, but if you are a child of the Most High God, you would know death is a beautiful experience. Think for a second, the few things that gives Satan power is you opening the door to fear. He smells fear and he knows what it look like. When God told Abraham to take his only son Isaac, whom he loved to the land of Moriah to be sacrifice as a bunt offering, Abraham didn't fear God, he walked in faith knowing God would be able to raise his son from the sting of death.

Today, I have a peace within my spirit that Irene is resting in the arms of the Lord. And I'm looking forward to meeting her again on the other side.

Do you believe you will see your love one again? Friend, you have a right to see your loves ones again because of what Jesus done on the cross, he took care of our sins through the cleansing of His precious blood. I am convinced that death was paid for on the cross.

Its time to stand to your feet child of God, and worship and praise your way through any dark valleys, and don't look at what's going on in you mortal bodies, God is able to bring healing to you. *"Weeping may endure for a night, but joy cometh in the morning"* (Psalm 30:5-7).

God says I'm going to, *"bestow on them a crown of beauty instead of ashes, the oil of joy instead of mourning, and a garment of praise instead of a spirit of despair. They will be called oaks of righteousness, a planning of the LORD for the display of his splendor"* (Isaiah 61:3).

CHAPTER TWO

Shaken By Cancer

"In the world you will have tribulation but be of good cheer, I have overcome the world" (John 16:33).

It has been a seven years since my friend Irene went home to be with the Lord. She made the trip that all of us will take someday; her time was just a little earlier than ours. The day of her death, I walk away from her bedside with great anger towards God. It never occurred to me that my day would come for me to battle this deadly disease called cancer.

August 13, 2011, I'd found a large lump in my right breast. In that moment, I thought to myself, surely it is just a cyst or large boil. The next day I phone my male gynecologist and told him about the lump I had discovered. He recommended I come in for a checkup. After examining me, the doctor broke the news to me gentle.   28.

"Mrs. Graham, you have two unknown large masses, one under your right arm and the other one is in your right breast." he said.

At that moment I could see the shock in his eyes as he sympathetically, referred me to the Solace clinic for a Diagnostic Breast Evaluation Mammogram; he said he could not give me any definitive diagnosis as to rather it was cancer or tumor. Immediately terror rocked my mind. Herbert and I were speechless; the news threw us for a loop.

The ugly word cancer keep racing back and forth in my mind, predicting its presence in my body. I started rebuking the thought by quoting my favorite Scripture.

"He was wounded for our transgressions, He was bruised for our iniquities; The chastisement for our peace was upon Him, And by His stripes we are healed" (Isaiah 53: 5-6). As I stood to walk out of the doctor's office Herbert held my hand and said, "Teresa, we will get through this too." I could see in his eyes he was scared.

Shaken By Cancer

The next morning, I walked into the Solace clinic with confidence

believing this doctor will not find anything but a tumor.

Instead, the medical doctor who performed the test confirmed with a

look of surety that a scan showed it was indeed cancer. I wanted to

jump off that table and run and hide under a big rock. I just could not

believe this could happen to me. I thought is this it for me, am I going

to dry up to bones, and be eaten alive like the cancer ate my friend

Irene. My eyes filled with tears as I glazed over to see the dark images

on the screen as the doctor explain his findings to me.

All I could think about was how horrible my friend death was

and how her body had deteriorated to a point she was just skin and

bones. The fear of cancer now chain my mind into thinking my time

has come to join my friend in glory.

Thoughts of leaving my family behind and dying so young

were very frightened to me. I had attempted to build my faith up by

quoting healing scriptures with fear attached to them, forgetting fear will eat my faith away like cancer.

Therefore, I had to come to a decision in my personal life to see myself healed. I knew if I wanted to beat the cancer, I would have to make God's word final authority in my life, and change my eating habits.

Prior to my diagnosis, I was very poor at eating the right so-called foods. I would eat sugar like there was no tomorrow. Not knowing that cancer cells loves sugar and it was known as a super food into making the tumor cells grow larger. Now who would ever think that cancer will be the thing to make me pay close attention to what I was feeling my body.

I started researching books on how to eat healthy in search to find the best healing remedies for my body. Therefore, in my research I found the one thing I love the most was bad for my health and that was sugar. Investigating the affect of sugar, I learned that sugar does pose a health risk in cancer patients.

Shaken By Cancer

Study shows from a research published through the pages of the

Journal proceeding of the

national Academy of sciences that it has been stated since 1923 tumor

cells uses a lot more glucose than normal cells. Dr. Thomas Graeber, a

professor of molecular and medical pharmacology, has investigated

how the metabolism of glucose affects the biochemical signals present

in cancer cells. In research published June 26, 2012, in the journal

Molecular Systems Biology, Graebar and his team of colleagues

demonstrates that glucose starvation—that is, depriving cancer cells

of glucose—-activates a metabolic and signaling amplification loop

that leads to cancer cell death as a result of the toxic accumulation of

reactive oxygen species.

When I began to understand the truth about sugar and how it

was affecting my body, I started erase sugar for my diet. I knew if I

was going to have a good chance be Didn't is deadly disease, I needed

to quickly start sugar cancellation.

Trust me when I tell you that my not eating sugar what the hardest thing I had to break, it was a battle within my mind. The file became hard because of my addiction for me years and this is why the fight was hard.

After about a month of reading books about sugar intake, I knew the sugar eating problem was a bad one and it was high time, I sent it packing.

On Thursday, I received a call from the doctors office nurse; she reviewed my biopsy results and said, "Mrs. Graham, the test shows that you do have cancer and it stage III breast cancer and its size is 3cm and we need to get you into our facility to see a doctor right away." The moment she uttered the word stage III breast cancer, fear gripped my soul. My knees got week as though someone hit me in my gut and I was out of breath. I set speechless at my desk in my office and tried to figure out what had just happened. My brain had lost its ability to discern between facts.

Soon, I found myself in a state of confusion even though I

heard a nurse clearly. The word cancel is always a fearful word because people usually associate it with sudden death. As I had mentioned earlier, my friend Irene lost her battle to stomach cancer and the devil wanted me to take the fight I am faced with would be lost to death.

Nevertheless, his fear attack ended it quickly. The words in my head started boldly shouted, "The devil is a liar! Not Me! I Shall Live and not die, and declare the works that the Lord has set before me."

However, I was determined not to allow that lie or the cancer rule my soul. Therefore, immediately I went into a fighting mode for my life. What challenged me, however, was the anger that I felt when I heard the word cancer. I felt terrible as a minister of the gospel and afraid for my future. Thoughts of taking chemotherapy and radiation was a great challenge for me. I knew the devil was here to test my faith in God. He wanted to see you did not really believe God would heal me or Will accept death as my final destiny.

"The devil is a Liar! Not Me!"

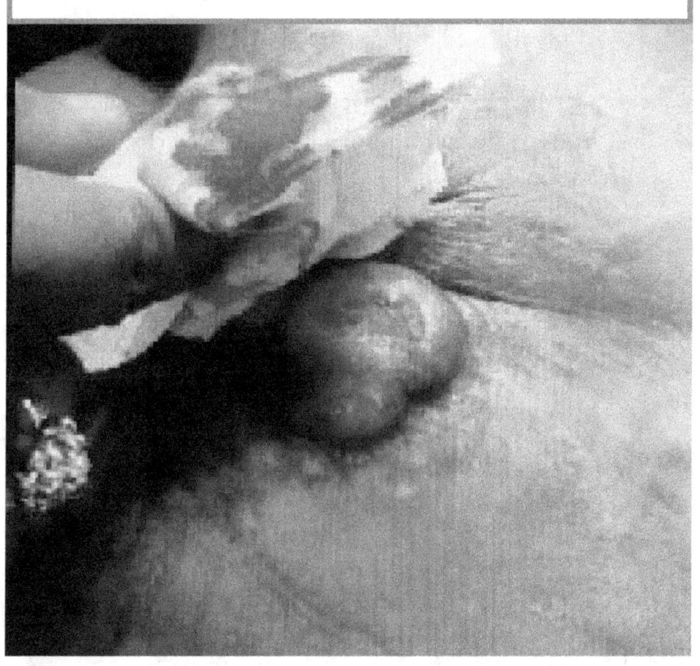

A Picture of changing the bandage from the tumors on my chest wall.

CHAPTER THREE

Healing The Mind

"Let this mind be in you which was also in Christ Jesus"

(Philippians 2:5).

Now that I was dealing with the cancer that griped my body, my mind started spinning. I had become confused and found myself asking God questions as to what was going on with my body. I was becoming angry with God for allowing my body to go through this battle, because over the months prior to my diagnosis, I'd been praying faithfully for people in various cities on the Daniel prayer line God had allowed as part of my ministry. I was happy, healthy, very content in life, and a woman who was on the move to do great things for the Lord. 36.

In fact, during 2010, I'd experience one of the most incredible times of my life. I founded Gospel Talk Television show which aired weekly on the Fort Worth Community cable channel.

I had self published several books, "Cultivate Me O' Jehovah, You Gotta Say Something, Break Mold Shape Me Lord, and a book on Daily Devotions. I tried to convince myself after losing my best friend things were going in the right direction. It looked like 2010 what's going to be an awesome year for me to blossom in the ministry and I thought to myself Life could not get any better than this!

Shockingly, cancer was on the scene to shake my faith beyond my wildest imagination. I thought how could I as a minister of the gospel stand in the pulpit and minister healing scriptures the people when I so desperately needed healing in my life... Time stood still as I cried on the floor. I really do not know how long I was kneeling, praying, and calling on the name of Jesus, but when I Finally did get, God gave me peace to know I was not going to die.

Healing The Mind

Friend, I had to align my mind with the word of God. When Jesus was being tempted in the wilderness, he knew he could not fight the devil with flesh and blood. He knew the only recourse that he had, what the Holy Word of God, by saying to the devil, "It is written…" instead of me lying down playing the victim letting cancer eat at my flesh and defeat me, I started praying, rehearsing in my mind, believing in my spirit, and decreeing and declaring that I'm healed in Jesus Christ name, every day. I will look in the mirror at my weak body and declare, "I shall not die, but live, and declare the works of the Lord" (Psalm 118:17).

Although I was overcome with emotion and ached at the thought of the evidence of cancer being in my body, I kept speaking on a daily basis healing Scriptures against those growing tumors believing they would dry up at the root and die. My faith and desperation caused me to make a trip to the cemetery I had never been to before.

I had heard about this anointed woman named sister Dodie Osteen who also had cancer. In her book, "Healed of Cancer," she talks a bout how the doctor met her husband in the lobby older hospital as he was visiting her the doctor delivered devastating news. He said that her husband, pastor, your wife has metastatic cancer of the liver. With or without chemotherapy, she has only a few weeks to live. He went on to say, "We can you treat her, but it will only slightly prolong her life."

Wow, what a blow from her doctor's Mouth speaking death over her life. I am sure that grim news shocked her inner core. However, the most important thing she told me in her book was how to develop a bulldog faith. She said in her book when she and her husband would drive by two cemeteries on their way to church she would personalize scriptures. Within moments, I found myself walking open down unknown graves in the cemetery declaring these words: Grave you have no problem over me, you have no place for my body today, I shall live and not die come I will not die prematurely   39.

He was wounded for our transgressions, he was bruised for our iniquities; the chastisement for our peace was upon Him, and by His stripes we were healed" (Isaiah 53:5).

After speaking boldly decreeing and declaring the Word of God for 20 minutes, I felt this energy shoot through my body as my faith level in God begin to rise up like a giant killer, and it was in that moment I knew God had healed my body from cancer.

I had become stronger, motivated, and more determined to fight like Dodie did, *"Fighting the good fight of faith"* (1 Timothy 6:12). I felt if God did it for her, surely he would heal me. I had placed my confidence in Jesus Christ and His word as being final authority in and yesterday, today, and forever." What the Scripture is saying, "Jesus Christ has never changed. What He did for Dodie He was going to do for me, and I was expecting God to totally heal my body!

Jesus gave His word for our protection. I knew from Scripture, He was wounded for our transgressions, He was bruised for our iniquities; The chastisement for our peace was upon Him, and by His stripes we are healed" (Isaiah 53:5-6).

I felt completely bathed and renewed in Jesus love, and His love made me feel as though I could conquer the world. I knew I had to stand on every promises of God, and resist the devil when he comes against my mind to steal the Word that has been planted into my heart. I knew I had to put up a shield of faith and refuse to allow the doctor's report to steal God's word out of my heart. I was willing and determine to hold fast to God's word until my victory came. That's why Philippians 4:6 says, "Do not fret or have any anxiety about anything" (AMP).

On the morning of my meeting with the breast surgeon, we discuss what the MRI results was and he reviewed with me the options he felt I had at that point. He had suggested a combination of chemotherapy and radiation after he remove one breast and some lymph nodes.   41.

Healing The Mind

As I sat straight up in my chair rehearsing the words of my doctor in my mind, I started praying as I turn to him saying, "I would like to have both breast removed to ensure this cancer will not come back years from now," I said.

"Mrs. Graham, there's no guarantee of your survivor rate even if you had both breast removed," he said sympathetically. In an attempt to pull my thoughts together blocking out what my doctor just said. I became convinced in my mind that death will not be my story anytime soon, because I knew God wasn't finish with me. *"Being confident of this very thing, that he which hath begun a good work in you will perform it until the day of Jesus Christ:"* (Philippians 1:6). As I looked into my doctor eyes, I could sense fear was in the inner core of his being and he did not know God sent a woman of faith to remain the doctors God is still a healer. I could "see in his eyes he had a look of concern and I wanted to prove to him and every doubter, God is a healer." I felt I needed to roll up my spiritual sleeves and get to work with the word of God.

The strangest thing beloved, I knew the devil was ready to use this cancer as a tool to beat me down physically and mentally, but I was determined to use God's word as a tool to defeat the attack cancer brought against my body. However, my doctors felt my chances might be great with 16 weeks of chemotherapy and six weeks of radiation and just maybe my survivor rate will be great.

On February 28, 2012, I awoke from nine-twelve hour surgery, there by my side stood, pastor Graham, and my two handsome sons smiling down at me as they stood over my bed. I was a little uncomfortable because there were tubes, oxygen tank, drainage bags and IV's still connected to my body. In walks the nurse, "Mrs. Graham, the doctor said your surgery went well, and your doctors will be in to speak with you in the morning. I will be your nurse for the entire time of your hospital stay" she said as she begin writing her name on the white board hanging on the wall in front of me. As I laid still trying to gather my thoughts, my eyes filled with blurriness glazed around the room slowly trying to adjust themselves to the bright lights of the radiating throughout the room. I was still a little groggy and daze, but hours later, I was sitting straight up in the hospital bed, acting like wonder woman, asking for solid food. I was hungry and thirsty and very determine to get my strength back so my stay at the hospital would be a short stay. Little did I know cancer would show its ugly presence months later.

The next morning my doctor was very shock to see me up and eating, he thought I would still be knocked out under the anesthesia, after having had a nine-twelve hour surgery. What they didn't know was, I had a little talk with the Lord before going into the surgery and I had another chat with Him when the surgery was over. My faith in God was a *"sure faith."* I went into the surgery expecting to get great results because I was the just and I lived my life by faith. As a minister of the gospel, God taught me six things about the characteristics of faith I think will bless you.

1. *Faith sees & hears.* The Bible says, "So then faith cometh by hearing, and hearing by the word of God" (Romans 10:17).

2. *Faith speaks.* The Bible says, "As it is written, I have made thee a father of many nations,) before him whom he believed, even God, who quickeneth the dead, and calleth those things which be not as though they were.

3. *Faith acts.* The Bible says, "For as the body without the spirit is dead, so faith without works is dead also" (James 2:26).

4. *Faith stands.* The Bible says, "Trust in the Lord with all thine heart; and lean not unto thine own understanding. In all thy ways acknowledge him, and he shall direct thy paths" (Proverbs 3:5-6).

5. *Faith rejoices.* The Bible says, "I will bless the Lord at all times: his praise shall continually be in my mouth" (Psalm 34:1).

6. *Faith receives.* The Bible says, "O give thanks unto the LORD, for he is good: for his mercy endureth for ever" (Psalm 107:1).

Also, faith needs someone to come in agreement with you because the Bible says, "Again, I tell you truly that if two of you on the earth agree about anything you ask for, it will be done for you by My Father in heaven. For where two or three gather together in My name, there am I in the midst of them" (Matthew 18:20).

Friend, where is your faith in God? He wants you to trust in him with all of your heart and lean not unto your own understanding, but in all your ways acknowledge him and he shall direct your path. God wants you to find someone with faith like yours who will not rehearse your demise but rehearse your healing today!

After surgery, I had blocked the pain mentally and even though I felt some pain radiating through my right arm and on the right side of my body, it wasn't that bad that I had to hit the morphine pump, because I had programmed my mind into thinking the pain didn't exist, and I didn't want the doctors or my family to think this C-word was going to kill me. Please understand, I did feel some pain after the surgery and if I had to rate the pain, I would say the pain from one to ten was about a seven.

Honestly, I can say for some strange unknown reason my body had always took pain very well. I remember when I gave birth to my last two babies, I was given a C-section and several hours after giving birth to them, I would be in the hallway of the hospital walking up and down the hallway like I was taking a stroll in the park on a hot summer day.

The funny thing about the whole thing is, I could never to this day explain to you how I was able to program my mind against pain. I would exercise my faith-filled words against anything attacking or attaching itself to my body and immediately the words I spoke would become evidence.

My doctor hospitalized me for over 24 hours for observation. He wanted to make sure there wasn't excessive bleeding or blood clots forming in my legs. God couldn't have given me a team of doctors and nurses who sincerely cared for my well being. They were sharp and keen to the type of treatment they felt would restore my body back to its normal state.

During my healing process, I did experience some slight discomfort and my right arm was numb for a while, but overall I had no major pain or bleeding from the surgery.

Healing The Mind

So, I decided to refused to receive the morphine in the drip

pump to flow through my veins. Please don't misunderstand me, the

doctors God had blessed me with were passionated about their work

and I'm sure they wanted me to be healed. But, my faith was in the

healing power of the creator who made heaven and earth.

There was a small knock at the door as this beautiful white

woman walked into the room announcing herself. I turned my head

towards the door glancing across the room as she walked over

towards my bed.

"Mrs.Graham, how are you feeling?" Feeling a little

lightheaded I managed to force a quick small smile. I rubbed my

fingers across my forehead saying, "I'm feeling fine, thanks for

asking."

I'm Sherree Bennett, with Baylor All Saints Medical Center

Breast Center and I come to give you a few items to help you with the

healing process and the doctors told me you had a successful surgery,"

she said smiling.

"I feel great Ms. Bennett."

"Well, you don't look like you've had surgery, you're such a beautiful lady" she said with a small grin on her face as she carefully reached into the big white paper bag pulling out two small pillows and a mastectomy camisole bra.

My eyes filled with excitement, I took the camisole bra as she handed it to me and I started examining it from the front to the back curious as to how will it fit perfectly against my flat chest. I notice after Ms. Bennett watched me for a few minutes fumbling with the camisole bra, she quickly started explaining and showing me different ways the camisole bra can fit to my flat chest and as I placed the bra on it felt comfortable to my skin. I noticed the camisole bra was design with two removable drain pouches to hold the drains after surgery and it also had two pockets for the breast form mastectomy prosthesis to fit into the front pocket of the vest. She also started explaining how I should care for the drains after she saw how pleased I was with the fitting of the camisole bra. She gave me information

Healing The Mind

about Joan Katz's Breast Center and the 1-1 Chemo Teaching which consist of teachings about, "How to live on chemotherapy." I was very happy to know that there's information provided for the patients and their family members after the patient has gone home to recover from surgery.

Within one month after leaving the hospital I was on the road to a speedy recovery taking chemo. I had a lot of questions that no one in my circle both friends and family couldn't answer. I had to endure everything without friends and neighbors. I'm sure there were support groups searches the surrounded by hope, I could have joined to help with my healing process. Instead, I decided I would rely totally on God the Creator to heal me.

I realized today, that there will be countless women who fought knowing what they knew as being normal Will never look the same in their mirror, because of what their Mirror reflects. Every day, my mirror reflects awful memories of the illness that came and rob me of my sexy breast, throwing me into an emotional fit.

50.

I had begin to develop low self-esteem, I didn't think that was beautiful anymore, and I secretly thought in my mind "how can a man still love me fully while looking at the disfigurement of my body." What happen to my being fearfully and wonderfully made by God. I knew what the scripture says in Psalm 139:14, where it says, "I will praise you, for I am fearfully and wonderfully made; Marvelous are your works, and that my soul knows very well.

Meaning God skillfully created me to be beautiful but yet my Mirror is displaying a woman I never knew. So now I'm left to figure out the new me and the purpose for this journey. I found my elf being driven by my faith in God during the course of each one of my chemo treatments, the treatment plan and the schedule times fit my daily life style, I didn't have to feel overwhelm and exhausted from the many visit to the doctors. Did depression try to creep into my life? yes, I found myself angry with God as his minister, I had become sad and fighting against the spirit of depression with the Scriptures as my daily medicine. Not realizing God had me in a place of isolation to break my will and bring about a healing that will confound my doctors mind. And while I was in the midst of the storm i had made a choice to let strengthen and heal my body from the crown of my head to the soles of my feet. I would lay across my bed many nights praying and reading Scriptures calling on the name of Jesus Christ. And each time I called on His name, how was expecting him to live up to his word, "But He was wounded for our transgressions, He was bruised for our iniquities: The chastisement for our peace was upon Him, And by His stripes we are healed" (Isaiah 53:5).

Beloved, that meant healing was mine when I release my faith to grab a hold of my healing. I was like a bull-dog and I was determine to get my healing from God and I had made a conscious heartfelt decision that I wasn't going to turn him loose until he healed me.

Now, during many treatments, I had an opportunity to meet some awesome women who fought a good fight of faith. I can truly say the health care providers we had provided the emotional support we needed to get through our chemo treatments. I thank the Lord everyday we have people in the medical field that love their job.

I've come to realize that I will fight is not in our flesh or olive blood like this scripture says in Ephesians 6:12, it's in the spiritual realm. We as believers have to rise up and say, "I'm going to hold onto your hand Lord until I see my healing." God has given you the power to put a stop to the enemy tries to flood your mind with on a daily basis. You must take authority over what you allowed to flood your mind. Your mind is a battlefield where are the enemy loves to set up camp.

Most of us don't give much thought to the devil's plots. Too often we plant in our minds its God's will for us to be sick. It's time for you to remember what scripture says, "Beloved, I wish above all things that thou mayest prosper and be in good health, even as that's so prospereth" (3 John 2).

Healing The Mind

I feel the praise right there! Glory be to God... He want you to prosper in every area of your life. So, make it a point to praise God when you arise to see his sun shine peering through your window pane in the morning.

Praise the Lord, we don't have to allow the enemy to invade our minds with doubt. Our great High priest went to heaven as a sacrifice on our behalf. We can be healed today! God has promised us if we put all of our trust in Him, He will give us perfect peace in our minds and uproot all those dead seeds that had us bound over the years. Open your mouth today and begin declaring you are healed in Jesus Christ name!

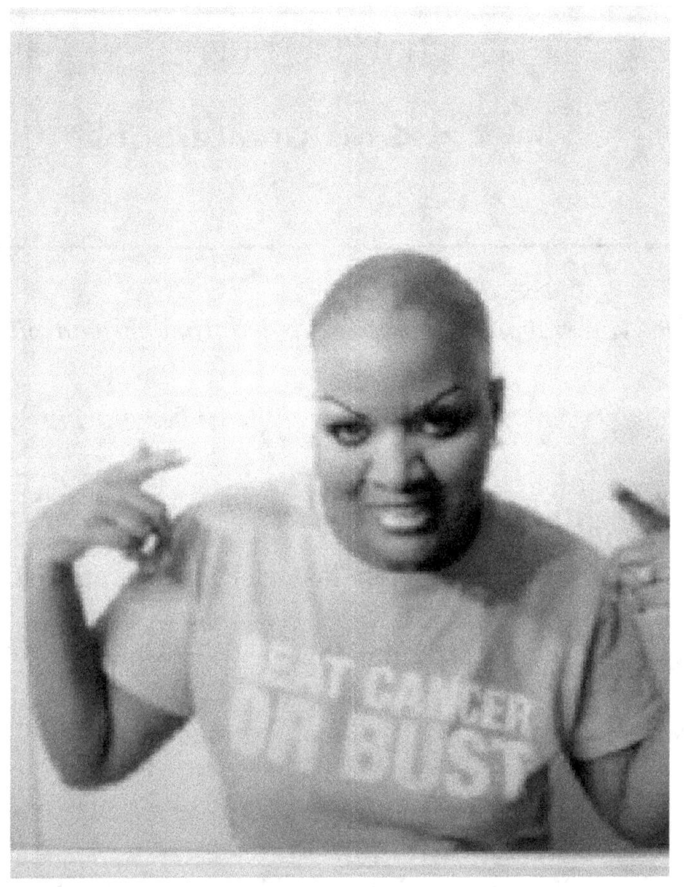

The Very First Day I Shaved My Head!

Beat Cancer Or Bust/Pink Tee-Shirt

Texas Oncologist Gave Me The Tee-Shirt

(September 2011)

CHAPTER FOUR

Why Did God Create Boob?

"That you may nurse and be satisfied from her consoling breast;

that you may drink deeply with delight from her glorious abundance"

(Isaiah 66:11).

When I was growing up in Miami, FL. I wanted to be a model with big beautiful breast to grab the attention of the men. As a little girl, I would at times make my breast by placing a pair of socks under my shirt to appear grown and sexy.

Finally, at the age of twelve puberty kicked in to cause my breast to grow to a noticeable size. They were full and round, I liked them, they had become a visual piece of objects for the world to see. Little did I know my well develop breast had a crucial role to play with bearing children.

At the very start of puberty I noticed a change in my body shape with the growth of pubic and body hair and a horrible menstruation that embarrassed the heck out of me in the middle of a school day. There wasn't any type of warning, it just decides to show up and make my life memorable, and trust me that day is still imprinted in my mind.

As I sat at my desk, blood started running down my legs and my classmates started laughing and poking fun at me until I started crying. They had placed me on the laughing block for weeks until I had enough and started fighting them back during recess.
I tried telling the teacher, I tried walking away and when that didn't work, I took matters in my own hands. I was known to kick some butts and from that moment my classmates respected me forgetting about my bleeding incident.

As for the development of my breast size, they had started as small buds at the age of ten and around 12 is when my breast was visible evidence of puberty.

Why Did God Create Boobs?

My breast made me feel like a little sex object, if you told me that my breast and I wasn't sexy, I would call you a liar! I was very young and foolish to think that God made my breast to be something other than breast feeding my children.

I now realize that God's plan was for me to us my breast to nurture my babies at the breast and to provide nourishment. In the book of Exodus 2:9 Pharaoh's daughter gave Mose to his mother asking her to "Take this child, and nurse it for me, and I will give the thy wages."

I was able to see from Scripture, God didn't just give us our beautiful breast to form our woman's figure, but to provide nourishment for our children. As we know breastfeeding is a biological function of our womanhood. When breastfeeding takes place it makes nursing and nurturing a feel-good feeling causing a bond between the mother and her child.

This bond is not only between the mother and her child, but your partner bonds with you when he touches, massages your breasts, it sends a spark stimulating to the nerves and your brain.

There, it triggers the release of a neurochemical called oxytocin from the brain's hypothalamus. This oxytocin stimulates the muscles in a woman's breast causing the milk to form.

I've come to realize that men are like the ape species obsessed with the woman breast. Now you ladies know, men are very visual and they notice every little feature on your body. You become a car on the car lot when they go looking for the features that a car has to offer. Men likes what they like, rather they are saved or not. The saying on the street is, "Bigger Is Better."

In my research, there are countless studies about boobs and personal preferences. The saying is, ***"Poor men like them big and Rich men like them small."*** Here's what the Song of Solomon had to say about the women breast.

"Your stature is like a palm tree, and your breasts are like its clusters. I say I will climb the palm tree and lay hold of its fruit. Oh may your breasts be like clusters of the vine, and the scent of your breath like apples" (Song of Solomon 7:7-8).

Why Did God Create Boobs?

It sounds like from scripture, ***King Solomon*** was a great lover of the woman breast because he makes more reference about the woman breast in other places in the Bible, if you read the whole book of Song of Solomon you will find some more erotic verses about the female breast. The way he talks about them in a seductive way.

Now ladies, I want you to put on the thinking cap for just a second, do you ladies see cats and dogs sucking on the breast for pleasure? The only time an animal suck on its mother's breast is when that mother is feeding its babe, and when that cub reaches a certain age, that mother pushes that cub away and that cub is left to defend for itself. It is my belief that men have incorporated women breast into their sex acts, turning them into more pleasurable sex toys.

It is a known fact that the breast does triggers men during their sex acts with their partner. You know, for a long time watching nature was never my thing, but the more I'm communicating with God in prayer, He is teaching me the order of His creation and how it operates.

We're superior beings, but yet we operate out of the order of God and become immune to sin with no regards to seeking Him for the correct way to live *His Divine Order.* I never paid attention to why God created women with boobs until my girls (boobs) was faced with stage III & IV breast cancer, and my sister had to remind me that I wasn't my *"boobs."*

I though for a second I was being punish for wanting to entice men with my full rounded breast, because Scripture does say, "Your sin will find you out" (Numbers 32:23). I was left feeling my sins came home to roost, but later found as facts, countless women were being diagnose with the C word.

The National Cancer Institute states, 12.4 percent of women born in the United States today will develop breast cancer at some time during their lives. The risk for breast cancer, however, is not the same for all women in a given age group. Research has shown that having a close male blood relative with breast cancer also increases a woman's risk of developing the disease.

Why Did God Create Boobs?

The Medline Plus states, breast cancer happens most often to men between the ages of 60 and 70. Now the risk factors for male breast cancer includes exposure to radiation, a family history of breast cancer, and having high estrogen levels, which can happen with diseases like cirrhosis or Klinefelter's syndrome.

After reading Medline Plus report, I now know Breast Cancer does not discriminate, there's this a not-for-profit patient advocacy organization who brings people together to educate the world about breast cancer in men its called, ***"The Male Breast Cancer Coalition."*** According to the American Cancer Society; an estimated 2,000 men will be diagnosed with breast cancer this year.

This was shocking and upsetting news to me that a man can get breast cancer and the percentage is on the rise. Ladies, make sure you have your man, sons, fathers, cousins, uncles, and grand-pa get checked by a doctor right away, it could save their lives. They too needs to have a self examination regularly checking their breast tissues behind their nipples, and they find something strange, they can get further testing at a hospital or their private doctor.

It is my prayers that this book is bringing awareness to its readers, because the knowledge is a powerful tool to the human race, it will empower men and women to take control of their health. There are all kinds of breast Cancer foundation out there to help educate men and women who are inspiring hope to those who was diagnosed with breast cancer. There was a time in past years, I lack knowledge of vital issues about to breast cancer and what early detection meant, but now, I want to read every piece of literature that's talking about breast cancer in hopes of bringing awareness to the human race. If I could play a role in helping save a life before this deadly disease hit its next victim, Count me in.

Faith Tried

In retrospect, my faith was tried beyond measure. Like many men and women who was diagnosed with the C word, I ran to God with a bulldog faith, believing in my heart, "I will not die but live, and declare the works of the LORD" (Psalm 118:17).

Why Did God Create Boobs?

As a minister of the gospel, I knew God had more work for me to complete before I say goodbye to this world. I had become determine to live out the rest of my years re-training mind mind and body on the right foods to consume, and what I found was helpful to my healing process. I started living to eat and not eating to live. I made sure to eliminate white sugar for my diet and add more water, herbs and veggies replace of Eden pork. I started a light exercise to improve my quality of life, light running and walking in place is what I did, but doing my appointments with chemotherapy and radiation I was able to perform any type of exercise routine because of feeling fatigue.

Another exercise I did was, I started feeding my mind and my soul daily with the word of God to increase my faith level during my journey of fighting breast cancer. God is a giver of faith. It is the "gift of God". Listen to what Scriptures Says, "For by grace are ye saved through faith; and that not of yourselves: it is the gift of God" (Ephesians 2:8). So we know that we can use the gift from the giver to ask for our healing. You can cause your faith to grow by daily exercise and it through the Bible. The person who doesn't exercise their faith will end up with poor faith. 2 Thessalonians 1:3 says, "We are bound to thank God always for you, brethren, as it is meet, because that your faith groweth exceedingly." This scripture is leaden you know that your faith can grow if you exercise it. You may say, "Teresa, how do I begin increasing my faith level to believe for my healing?" Good question, I'm glad you ask.

First step is, you have to begin where you are today. No one starts at the top of the ladder without first climbing from the bottom of the ladder. Make a habit to start a daily plan to read five faith scriptures in order to exercise your faith in God and pretty soon you will have developed a bull dog faith. **Never give up! You will get there!**

CHAPTER FIVE

Cancer With A Vengeance

"That the trail of your faith, being much more precious than gold that perisheth, though it be tried with fire, might be found unto praise and honour and glory at the appearing of Jesus Christ:"

(1 Peter 1:7).

It's 9 P.M. on a Saturday night, I noticed some small tumors growing on my right chest area where the surgical scar was. I thought to myself it's probably an affection from the surgery, so I didn't think twice about it, I just went to sleep. I thought I could call my findings into the doctor next day, and he will prescribe me some antibiotics over-the-counter, but reoccurrence was on the scene to rock my world once again.

In January 2013, I was diagnosed with a recurrence of invasive ductal carcinoma stage for breast cancer after the biopsy showed the cancer was back. I was given an appointment to visit my chemo doctor and during my visit blood was drawn before the nurse and escorted me into the exam room.

In walks Dr. Pham, who's my cancer oncologist. I noticed when she walked in the exam room she had this certain look of concern on her face. The first question she asked me after greeting me was, "Are you afraid to die?" As stood in front of me waiting for an answer.

"No" I said.

Immediately after I said no there was this puzzle look on her face as she walked over to the stool in front of her computer, "Tell me why" she asked as she sat crossing her legs.

"Dr. Pham, I have faith that God will heal me, and I know a man named Jesus" I said. Her concern gaze told me, she didn't think I would live long. She stood to check my lungs and said, "The cancer has upgraded from a stage III to stage IV."

Cancer With A Vengeance

I looked her in the eyes and said, "What does that mean?"

She grabbed my test results looking down at them she said, Mrs. Graham, your CT scan is showing that the cancer is in both of your lungs, and we see some spots in the liver and the right breast," she said.

After the reading of my test results, she held up my test results for me to read them. There it was plain as day cancer in my body once again making it self known in my world.

I took a deep breath before asking, "Dr. Pham, Will I have to take chemo again?" She nodded saying, "No, it didn't respond well the first time, so we will try you on a chemo drug called Xeloda which will be a pill form." Following her response, my next question was, take my hair out again and how long did I have to pop these pills?

Dr. Pham, almost knocked the breath out of my body with her response.

"Teresa come you have to be on Xeloda for the rest of your life, and it's no guarantee the drug will work because your body will at some point in time become immune to the drugs which will cause the cancer to attack your body" she said with compassion. I could tell by the tone of the voice she was in fear for my life. So now the cancer was back, and I was left once again to dig deeper into the word of God exercising my bull-dog faith. I was just placed into the furnace that was heated seven times hot. I had to exercise my faith in God like the three Hebrew boys who was believing God that they would escape the fiery furnace. Dr. Pham, had just handed me a death sentence without a date.

I looked up and said, "I have faith God will heal me." And I picked up my things to leave. As I left the office, I knew without a doubt god was going to show his healing power through my body and destroy that cancer that has invaded my body without my permission.

The next day I received a phone call from Texas Oncologist nurse for Dr. Parks. She says, "Hello Ms. Graham, Dr. Chi Pham, would like for you to see Dr. Park, who is our radiation Oncologist. When would you like to make the appointment?"

Cancer With A Vengeance

I thought to myself, never.

"Whatever days you have available will be fine with me" I said.

"Will tomorrow at 9. A.M., work for you Mrs. Graham" she ask.

"Yes," I said. "Okay, Ms. Graham, we will see you in the morning, and make sure to bring your picture ID and proof of your insurance" she said before hanging up the phone.

I sat calmly in my chair gazing out the window, "Surely God you are going to get the glory out of this in the end." Even though I didn't want to fight again, I decided to roll up my spiritual sleeves and told the devil, "A fight you want, a fight you will receive, your arms is to short to box with God."

I found myself in my prayer closet every night rising before the sun calling on the name of Jesus Christ for my healing. Although I was overcome with emotion and ached at the thought of dying at an early age. Thoughts of ending my life played back and forth in my mind, it was a passing thought that stems from the news of having cancer again.   70.

I had begin to feel isolated and hurt wishing this was just a bad dream

playing a bad prank on me. The pain had felt overwhelming and

depression tried to grip my mind and death was beginning to look

good to the ending of my problem.

But, a small still voice said, "Teresa, your life isn't yours to take, I

have work for you to do." And from that day forward, I rose up like a

trooper and decree and declare, *"I shall not die, but live, and declare

the works of the LORD"* (Psalm 118:17). After realizing God still

have work for me to do, I never allowed the spirit of suicide to attach

it self to me. I can truly say, this second battle with breast cancer

changed my life forever.

I was left to take Isaiah 61:3 personal where it says,

"To all who mourn in Israel, he will give a crown of beauty for ashes,

a joyous blessing instead of mourning, festive praise instead of

despair. In their righteousness, they well be like great oaks that the

LORD has planted for his own glory."

Cancer With A Vengeance

I held on to this Scripture for inner-healing. And, I knew someday the Lord would allow me to release my healing journey through the pages of this book, ***"You're Not Your Boobs."*** God has given me beauty for ashes, he has shown his love through this whole journey and he has empowered me to help others to know that the battle isn't theirs, it's the Lord's.

The next 16 weeks was just filled with being on the radiation table from Monday - Friday for 15 minutes a day. I had an amazing 16 weeks taking radiation, each treatment was a joy to my soul. The Lord sent angels in the form of nurses to care for me. I remember laying on the table looking into the ceiling listening to the sound of Christian music play softly through out the exam room.

I felt like I had just died and went to heaven, the nurse had such an angelic voice, she made me forget why I was laying on the table. She would bend over singing in my ears at the same time of zapping me with the radiation machine. She made my time spent there a memorable one. I would jump off the table and starting dancing to the music and praising God with them, and one of the nurses walked

in and saw us dancing and said, "This is the type of party I like." We

turned that exam room out that day with a praise dance!

As weeks passed by, my oncologist was very please about the

outcome of my treatments. And the last day, there was the ringing of

the victory bell which is a significant moment signaling the end of

treatment and the beginning of being cancer free. Everyone gathered

around me in the hallway, clapping and applauding, as I pull the string

making a joyful sound of completion of my radiation treatments,

everyone rushed over giving me a hug and one of the ladies handed

me a signed certificate to confirm the cancer was destroyed.

A week later, I applied for my medical disability and was

immediately granted to receive a monthly check. I was happy about

receiving the check, but I'd rather work. I wasn't able to work on

anyone's job because of my medical condition that is expected to last

at least five years-or more. I still had the chemo-port in place later

removing it after ten months.

Cancer With A Vengeance

My oncologist said she had no further use for it and said its up to me rather I want to have it remove. I had it in for a long time and it was hard to draw blood from because the scar tissue was building up around it, and the only reason I kept it in because I don't have good veins in my arms. Today, I wish I would have left the chemo port in because every doctors appointment requires lab work and sticking my veins comes along with the territory not to mention I hate needles.

I felt a little tenderness at the port site for a few days up to two weeks after my doctor removed it. During my recovery, I started writing songs which led me to record my first single, "Second Chance." This song came about one day while laying in my family room on the sofa having a conversation with God. The thought of Him given humankind a second chance when He sent His Son to die on the tree which is the cross for us was mind blowing.

So, I would lay on the sofa and hum the lyrics out aloud and listening as the song took shape. I later called my oldest son Charles, who's also was musically incline, we recorded the rough draft in his home studio before recording the complete song at Sessions Works

studio. The song went on to be nominated as best Female Gospel

Artist & best Female Christian Artist with Indie Music Channel

Awards, based out of Los Angels California. What a blessing!

I didn't let the chemo-port stop me from going into the studio

to record my songs, in fact, I spoke to the chemo-port and told it,

"You will become my friend and not harm me." I would speak to the

chemo pills and tell them the same thing. I was determine to live and

not die. I never liked taking the chemo pills, they would have my feet

and hands blacker than my shoes, I'm a light skinned girl looking like

I had just rub black tar over my body. I thought, surely there has to be

another way my body can receive the healing it needed.

One day while sitting in my office at my desk praying. I had

just taken the four pills I was prescribe by my doctor to take, and was

soon to take another four before going to bed, which would be a total

of eight pills a day, when all of a sudden in a vision, I saw my spirit

leave my body, followed by a still small voice saying,

Cancer With A Vengeance

"Don't you take another chemo-pill, go to the health-food store and pickup these herbs and pray over them and replace them with the chemo-pills."

 I immediately obeyed the voice of the Lord and today, I am healed. I've been taking CT-Scans, every three months which moved to every six months, looking forward to hear Dr. Pham say from her lips, "We're moving your appointments to once a year." Now that's when you know you doing great!

"Trust in the LORD with all your heart and lean not on your own understanding; In all thy ways acknowledge him, and he shall direct thy paths" (Proverbs 3:5-6).

CHAPTER SIX

Have Faith In God To Heal You

"So then faith cometh by hearing, and hearing by the word of God"

(Romans 10:17).

I remember one day asking God to increase my faith, I didn't know my faith was about to be tried beyond measure. Listen to what the Lord told the apostle in Luke 17:6 after they asked for an increase in their faith, "If you have faith as a mustard seed, you can say to this mulberry tree, "Be pulled up by the roots and be planted in the sea, and it would obey you." Look how powerful a small seed of faith will do for your big situation. Small faith will heal you!

Having stage IV breast cancer was a big huge mountain, and I needed my faith increase with the big faith God had increased in my life over the years. I always tell people, everything I have, is because I allow faith to birth things into the natural, and not let what my *natural, eyes* may see, or dictate to me what my *faith eyes* says I can have.   77.

Have Faith In God To Heal You

I've learned to trust God when I couldn't see my way out. He has always been there, waiting to rescue me from the storm. The things I saw God do through my life since walking in faith, will cause an atheist to get saved.

Some people may think that I'm crazy for saying this, but I'm glad to have gone through breast cancer, and been healed by God, because it just shows once again, the God that we serve is still on the throne. If the question was asked, "Would I want to go through the fight again? "No!" I would rather go jump off a bridge than to go through this again. I strongly believe my battle against this deadly disease wasn't about me, it was about the birthing of this book as a tool to help build others faith in God.

I could have played the victim, walking around saying, "Oh God, why me" but I chose to be the victor with my story, giving God some glory.

Did I question my faith walk with God during the healing process, "Yes I did!"

There was a point during my treatments I had passed by the mirror and took a peek at the big cancerous tumors, over taken the right side chest, they were busting open like an open flower for the world to see, blood and pus leaking from the tumors through out the day was enough for anyone to lose their mind.

At one point, I did entertained the thought of dying because of the way the big cancerous sores was eating at my body. My *fleshy eyes* was fighting with my *faith eyes* saying, "Where is your *faith eyes* now and what are you allowing your eyes to believe? Don't you see those big nasty tumors all over your body girl, eating away at your flesh, you are surely going to die! The voice just kept pounding over and over in my mind as my eyes kept seeing these words in big bold letters. "Stop kidding yourself, people have died with stage IV breast cancer, and you young lady, will soon join them!"

Now it was time for my faith eyes to speak to my lying *fleshly eyes* by saying, "Look here *fleshly eyes,* you've had your chance to speak and try to convince me that death is my tomorrow, but now its time for me to tell you what I see through my faith eyes by using the Word of God to back me up.

The Bible says, "So faith comes by hearing, and hearing by the word of God" (Romans 10:17). **Fleshly eyes, the** Bible says, "Jesus was wounded for my transgressions, He was bruised for my iniquities; the chastisement for my peace was upon Him. And by His stripes I'm healed" (see Isaiah 53:5). And **fleshly eyes,** "All sickness is not unto death, but for the glory of God" (see the account of Lazarus, John 11:1-4).

So, you see fleshly eyes, the sickness that attached it self to my body didn't have death as its final result, instead, it demonstrated His deity in an undeniable way. Stop talking!
I had to stop Mr. Fleshly Eyes, from painting the wrong picture in the attic of my mind, even though the evidence was there for the world to see, my faith eyes remained focused on God's healing power, and I

strongly believe today, I'm healed because of my faith in God, I work the Word of God, I believed the Word of God and it was God's Will for me to be totally healed from breast cancer.

The Scriptures says, "Death and life are in the power of the tongue, And those who love it will eat its fruit" (Proverbs 18:21). I made a conscience decision to live my life to the fullest and not let the words of my mouth ensnare my future. I didn't get here over night, I had to read the Word of God, see the Word of God, believe the Word of God, and speak the Word of God into manifestation.

I believe once you know your God-given rights through the Word of God, you can lay hold on them by speaking it into existence. The steps to recovery is never easy, and yes, there will be days you will want to give up and throw in the towel, if you trust in the lying fleshly eyes. But just know, healing belongs to you and it's yours for the taking.The same God healed me will be the same God to heal you. "For there is no partiality with God" (Romans 2:11). I know this Scripture is talking about a person's Salvation where Peter therefore said (as noted in the question), "Truly I perceive that God is not a respecter of persons," meaning (as indicated by other Bible translations of Acts 10:34 that God does not show any partiality or favoritism with respect to who could be saved through faith in Christ that both Jews and Gentiles who believed in Christ were now to be accepted as His followers.

I'm just saying that in all things, God does love and treats us the same. Never give up on God when you find your faith being tried by trials and tribulations. As the believer lives by faith, God continues to work in your favor and heal your body from any type of sickness. Always remember your mind have to lined up with the powerful Word of God, by transforming by the renewing of your mind in the way you see yourself in God. "Is there anything to hard for LORD?" (Genesis 18:3).

Let us think carefully about the power we now have on the inside of us. We have the power to uproot all those lies the devil has sown in our lives and against our bodies.

If God created the heavens and the earth, surely He can heal your body that's made of clay. "In the sweat of your face you shall eat bread till you return to the ground, For out of it you were taken; for dust you are, And to dust you shall return" (Genesis 3:19).

Every human being flesh will have their day to return back to the earth in which they came. Death is not a bad thing, I think people just fear the unknown part of death. Apostle Paul makes this profound statement about death in 2 Corinthians 4:8; "We are confident yes, well pleased rather to be absent from the body and to be present with the Lord." These Scriptures shows you and I where we will go when we leave this earth. Hallelujah! Glory Be To God!

I believe we as God's children need to embrace death and not let the fear of dying grip our inner-man. We can't be to attached to this world that we want to make it our home. Listen to what 1 Peter 2:11-12 says about this world being our home, "Friends, this world is not your home, so don't make yourselves cozy in it. Don't indulge your ego at the expense of your soul. Live an exemplary life among the natives so that your actions will refute their prejudices. Then they'll be won over to God's side and be there to join in the celebration when he arrives." Keep The Faith!

"What does it profit, my brethren, if someone says he has faith but does not have works? Can faith save him? 15 If a brother or sister is naked and destitute of daily food, 16. And one of you says to them, "Depart in peace, be warmed and filled," but you do not give them the things which are needed for the body, what does it profit? 17. Thus also faith by itself, if it does not have works, is dead" (James 2:14-26).

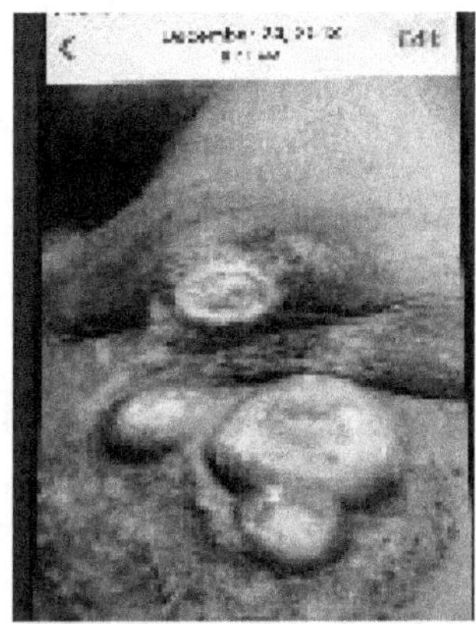
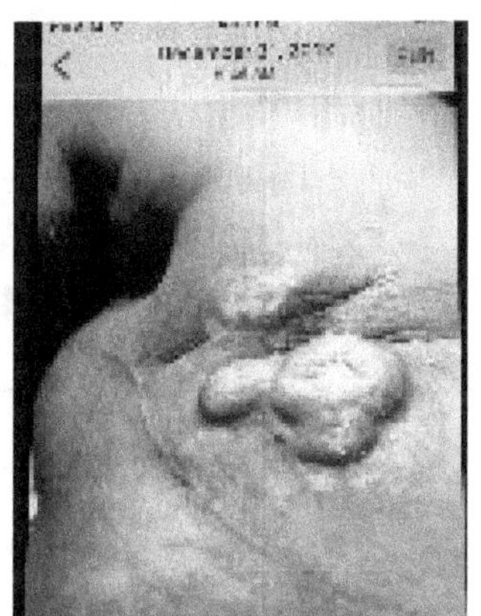
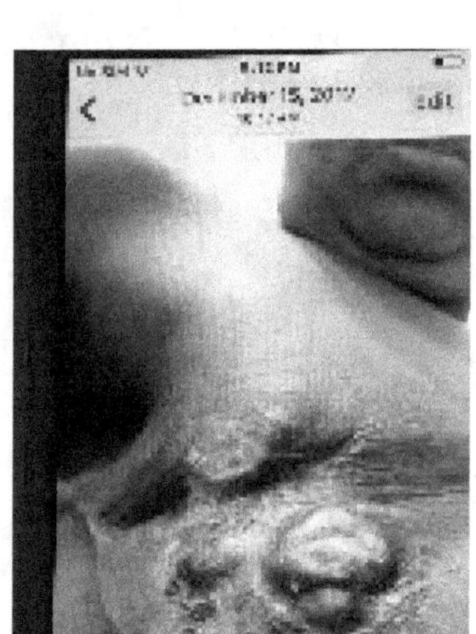
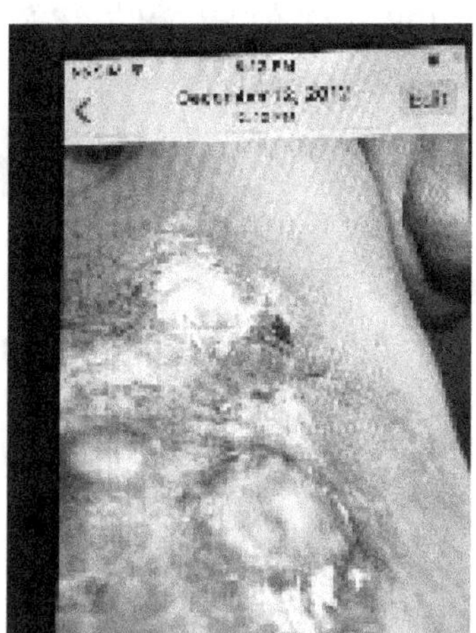

Pictures I took with my iPhone.

December 12 - December 31, 2012

CHAPTER SEVEN

Take A Spiritual Dose Everyday

"Finally, brethren, whatever things are true, whatever things are noble, whatever things are just, whatever things are pure, whatever things are lovely, whatever things are of good report, if there is any virtue and if there is anything praiseworthy—meditate on these things" (Philippians 4;8).

I had to learn the importance of taken a daily dose of the Word of God daily. **Spiritual medicine** vs **Conventional medicine** was far better for my soul and spirit-man.

I would often times set in my office gazing out the window with the chemo pills shaken in my hands, as I spoke Bible verses over them because my faith in God was to a point I needed those pills to realize I had divine authority over them.

Jesus said, "Behold, I give unto you power to tread on serpents and scorpions, and over all the power of the enemy: and nothing shall by any means hurt you" (Luke 10:19). That includes the chemo pills, God gave me power to tread upon and they would cause no harm to my body. Be careful what you hear when you are fighting for your life, you must be willing to do whatever it takes to survive. It is God's will that we be in good health.

"Beloved, I wish above all things that thou mayest prosper and be in health, even as thy soul prospereth" (3 John 2). That simply means, "When the enemy starts speaking sickness to you" get rid of it immediately. You may say, "Teresa, what can a person do when she or he is sick? My advice to you is to recite the promises of God until you see and feel your health be restored. When I fought for my life, I didn't see death from cancer was going to be the reason for my demise.

So, I was determined to eat the Word of God, morning, noon and night. I was determine to get my healing, in-spite of what it look like, feel like, or sound like, healing was mine, and I wasn't going to

turn to the Word of God loose, until He healed me. I believe we all

have some type of cross that we must bear, and we all will deal with

life on a different scale. What may work for you, may not be the right

solution to solve my issues, but you can bet your bottom dollar, If you

work the Word of God it will work for you no matter how bleak the

situation appears to be, you need to understand that the Word of God

does work if you work the Word!

<u>Scriptures For Your Thoughts</u>

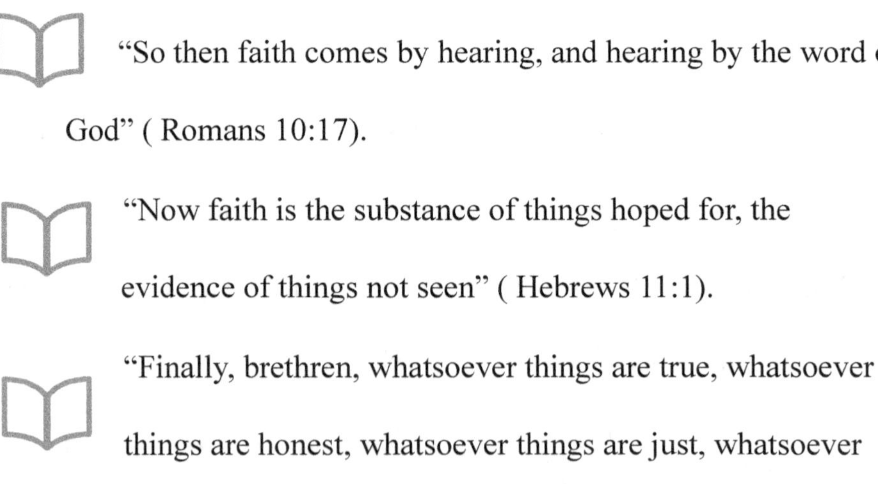

"So then faith comes by hearing, and hearing by the word of God" (Romans 10:17).

"Now faith is the substance of things hoped for, the evidence of things not seen" (Hebrews 11:1).

"Finally, brethren, whatsoever things are true, whatsoever things are honest, whatsoever things are just, whatsoever things are pure, whatsoever things are lovely, whatsoever things are of good report; if there be any virtue, and if there be any praise, think on these things" (Philippians 4:8).

"I shall not die, but live, and declare the works of the LORD" (Psalm 118:17).

"What shall we then say to these things? If God be for us, who can be against us?"

But he was pierced for our transgressions, he was crushed for our iniquities; the punishment that brought us peace was on him, and by his wounds we are healed" (Isaiah 53:5).

"Trust in the LORD with all your heart and lean not on your own understanding; In all your ways acknowledge him and he shall direct your path" (Proverbs 3:5-6).

"They will fight against you but will not overcome you, for I am with you and will rescue you, declares the LORD" (Jeremiah 1:19).   89.

Take A Spiritual Dose Everyday

These were some of the Scriptures I used as daily medicine. I would speak them two to three times a day. I would take communion twice a day after quoting my favorite Scriptures.

Never let the C word shape your mind into believing you will die. Twice Paul said to every believer to put on the full armor of God….the belt of truth (which deals with the covering of the heart) …the shield of faith (which is protection against any fiery darts of the enemy) and lastly the helmet of Salvation (which protects the mind)..Wow!

Look at the great protection we as born-again believers have to look forward to. Child of God, all you have to do is walk in that God-given authority and tell that cancer, "In the name of Jesus Christ, leave my body now!" And that cancer has to obey if it's the will of God for you to be healed. You must understand that the authority was given to you to destroy sickness, but you have to know your right.

Stop allowing the negative report of the C word kill what little faith you have. When faced with this deadly disease, this is the time you roll up your spiritual sleeves and run into the boxing ring with your gloves full of authority and power. Can I leave you with a small suggestion? My suggestion to you is that you fine you a good church or a good support group who knows the importance of prayer, people who would touch and agree with you on a daily basis, and help activate your faith. You must on a regular basis cultivate your faith with our heavenly Father, so that your faith will become strong against any voices that may try and speak negative words to get you discourage. Don't let the C word take root in your spirit-man. If you have a church family you see or talk to on a regular week, have them come over and break bread with you.

I was strong in my faith walk until I didn't need or sought a support group, all I wanted to do was be by myself to pray and read the Bible, automatically I knew God would give me the answer to my prayer, and He did!

Hair Cutting Day

I remember the very first day, I picked up a pair clippers to shave my hair, tears flood my cheeks, as I looked in the mirror at my reflection, praying this was just a sick nightmare or some sick joke. Only to find, it was cold reality I was forced to live. After the initial shock, I started screaming to the top of my lungs, "This is a war cry." Even though I saw shaving my head as another hit in the gut from this demon call cancer, I was willing to go through the fight because, I knew my redeemer lives, and I was going to watch Him get the victory from this. Some people have mistakenly concluded that God doesn't heal his people anymore, that was for the old time 2,000 years ago.

We as God's children need to understand Satan's weapon. He loves to blind the unbelievers, "If our gospel is veiled, it is veiled to those who are perishing, in whose case the god of this world has blinded the minds of the unbelieving, that they might not see the light of the gospel of the glory of Christ, who is the image of God"

(2 Corinthians 4:3-4).

And how do he do that? Through ignorance, unbelief and you not have the full knowledge of who you are in Christ Jesus.

Bottom line: Satan will have you for lunch, if you don't know who you are in God. If you choose to trust God in the middle of the fight, you will walk away victoriously. Even if you survive a bad fight, you will have a story to give God some glory. Do not allow what you see in the mirror cause you to lose hope in God. I can assure you that, "For the weapons of our warfare are not carnal, but mighty through God to the pulling down of strongholds;
(2 Corinthians 10:4).

Each experience has its own pain that pushes us to trust God. Just know beloved, He will give you what you need to survive the fight. It takes faith to let go and let God. The greatest tragedy is that people forget that God created them, and He knows what they need before they ask Him. Peter says, "God careth for you."

Take A Spiritual Dose Everyday

In Ephesians 3:20 Apostle Paul says that God is "able to do exceeding abundantly beyond all that we ask or think, according to the power that works within us." We can rest assure that inner power flows from God and is the basis of what we need to be healed.

From the very beginning of my hair cut, I'd experienced an incredible range of emotions. One moment I was ready to fight. The next moment, I wanted to throw in the towel. I had confess for years my faith in God, its easy to do when life is smelling like roses, but when the adversity shows up, what would your praise do then. Quickly you will find out how strong your faith is in the God you said you love.

As I mentioned in the last chapter, the steps to recovery is never easy, and yes, there will be days you will want to give up and throw in the towel, that's if you trust your fleshy eyes. Just know, healing belongs to you and it's yours for the taking.

The same God healed me will be the same God to hear you. "For there is no partiality with God" (Romans 2:11).

I know this Scripture is talking about a person's Salvation where Peter therefore said (as noted in the question), "Truly I perceive that God is not a respecter of persons," meaning (as indicated by other Bible translations of Acts 10:34 that God does not show any partiality or favoritism with respect to who could be saved through faith in Christ that both Jews and Gentiles who believed in Christ were now to be accepted as His followers.

I pray this book is helping somebody, I can only share my healing experience as a tool to help in your road to being healed. You have to know, God wants you healed and the devil wants you dead.

What do you want?

Words For Meditation

In the beginning God created the heaven and the earth. And the earth was without form, and void; and darkness was upon the face of the deep. And the Spirit of the God moved upon the face of the waters" *(Genesis 1:1-2).*

Take A Spiritual Dose Everyday

The Lord is my shepherd; I shall not want. He maketh me to lie down in green pastures: he leadeth me beside the still waters. He restoreth my soul: he leadeth me in the paths of righteousness for his name's sake. Yea, though I walk through the valley of the shadow of death, I will fear no evil: for thou art with me; thy rod and thy staff they comfort me. Thou preparest a table before me in the presence of mine enemies: thou anointest my head with oil; my cup runneth over. Surely goodness and mercy shall follow me all the days of my life: and I will dwell in the house of the Lord for ever. (Psalm 23: 1-6).

<u>*Note Taking*</u>

____

____

____

____

____

____

Write Down The Very First Day You Was Diagnose With Cancer

Time: ——————————— Date: ———————————

What Are Your Feeling Right Now?

Is There Anyone In Your Family Had Cancer?

Yes ————No ————

How Strong Is Your Faith In God?

____

____

Who Will Be Your Support Group?

____

____

____

____

How Much Sugar Intake Do You Consume A Day?

____

____

Do You Exercise Daily?

Yes————- No ————-

Do You Have Someone To Drive You To The Doctors?

____

____

____

____

<u>Are You Ready To Fight The Good Fight Of Faith?</u>

____

____

____

____

<u>Write Down Your Favorite Scripture From The Bible</u>

____

____

____

____

____

____

Are You Mad With God?

What Is Your Hobbies?

How Many Children Do You Have?

____

____

____

____

Did You Like Your Doctors And Nurses?

____

____

____

How Long Did You Take Chemo, Radiation?

____

____

____

____

What Type Of Cancer Was You Diagnose With?

____

____

____

____

Do You Have The Support Of Your Family And Friends?

Yes————————————————-No———————————-

Can You See Yourself Writing Book To Help Someone?

Yes————————————No————————

Write Down A Special Memory You Had During Your Battle

____

____

____

____

____

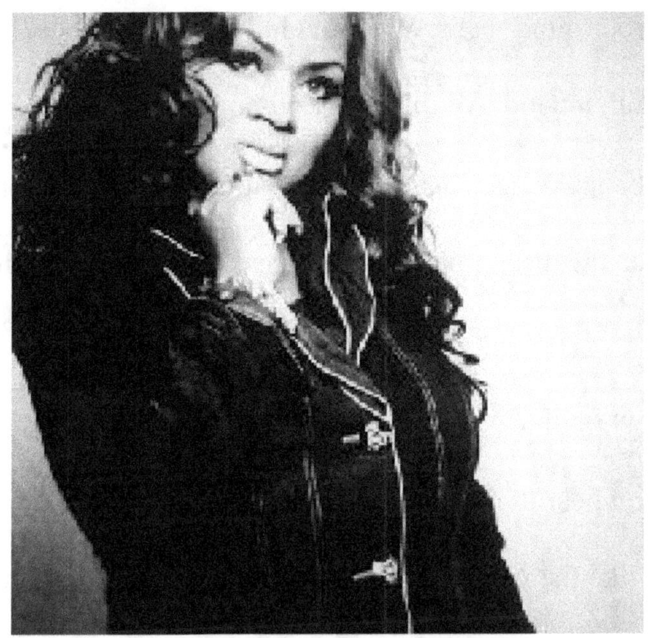

Dr. Teresa A. Graham's Personal Note To You.

I write to you as a friend who has battle stage III & stage IV breast cancer. I wanted to encourage you through this book not to give up the fight because the fight is not yours, but it's the Lord. You are strong, and you are powerful and you are blessed to have a story to give God some glory.

Friend, you must understand, you are uniquely endowed with beauty that will never forgotten. Breath in the love and grab a hold to your future, and learn to turn those lemons into lemonade, try to focus by keeping your mind on the Word of God which will cause you to plant your faith in God. All things are possible when you believe in the God of the universe. You are on the path to total healing, and you must lay aside the disappointments and make a decision to finish the race.

I know firsthand the hurt and pain that comes into your inner-man when you hear that C word flowing from your doctors lips. It feels almost like the world as suddenly stop moving, but your heart keeps bleeding. But I want to challenge you to start reading the Bible as daily medicine, I promise you, you will find peace, joy and happiness. Now you have to realize it may take sometime before you see your healing. You have to still praise Him in advance.

We must line our spoken words up with the Word of God. There's power in your tongue, "Death and life are in the power of the tongue: and they that love it shall eat the fruit thereof" (Proverbs 18:12).

My question to you is, "What do you want?" Death or life?

Once God's Word is birth in our heart, it releases the ability of God, so, whatever you do, never confess that you have cancer because you will become a product of what you spake into the atmosphere.

I made a decision to never own cancer as being a part of my life, I rejected it the very moment I heard the word cancer flowing from my doctor's lips. The evidence was there big as day, but my faith wouldn't allow me to receive what my fleshly eyes was seeing.

Some people might say, "Hey, I might as well get my house in order because I'm going to die from this cancer." You right! You will die, because you've just stamped your own death certificate.

<u>"JUST DIED."</u>

Always remember to watch your tongue and what you allow to escape your mouth, because it will become your grave, and don't let the spirit of fear or doubt take a seat at your table. Rebuke them now. Lets make your mind up that you aren't going to let him deposit fear into your heart.

Its time to make your mind up from this day forward that you aren't

going to let him deposit fear into your heart.

That means you will have to stay focus on the healing power

of Jesus. He says, *"My yoke is easy, and my burden is*

light" (Matthew 11:30).

<u>My daily regiments</u>

I started reading this book called, **<u>Dead Doctors Don't Lie,</u>** written

by ***Dr. Joel D. Wallach & Dr. Ma Lan.*** I ran across some information

that rocked my world. They were talking early symptom of selenium

deficiency in older human is the appearance of "liver spots" or age

spots. Than they were talking about how the Chinese for 5000 years

used **<u>Shark Cartilage and Shark Liver Oil</u>** to treat cancer, and their

recommendation for daily usage was 70 grams per day.

I don't have to tell you I drop everything to run to the health

food store and obtain those herbs to place in my daily regiment. I was

willing to try the moon if that would have brought about healing.

"Well, Teresa, I thought you said you live by faith."

Yes, you can have all the faith in the world, but if you don't put that action behind it, the Bible says, ***"Its dead."***

Lets make something clear, just because you have faith it will not automatic deliver you out of your problems. It is a known fact that cancer is an uncontrolled group of cells that kills the function of normal cells. So, it would be wise to maintain a healthy nutrition to help fight the cancer.

I was blessed not to have diarrhea or constipation during the days I received chemotherapy. I was told that many of the patients had side-effects, developing sores in their mouth and on their tongue. I thank God I was blessed not to have experience that side during my treatments. I did have to take the shots to boost my white blood cell count after a chemotherapy treatment.

Mastectomy Bras

I was fitted for a bra to wear the breast prosthetic until my reconstructed surgery was completed. These breast prosthetic bra shapes are designed to suit most contemporary, modified radical surgical techniques, where less breast tissue is removed.

I really liked them, no one knew I had fake boobs under my clothes but me, I tried on several occasion to get the silicone implants, my body would reject them. I would have break outs and high fevers to a point I was rapidly losing weigh. They were removed and now in October 23, 2017, I will have my final surgery, the DIEP flap, it involves the use of lower abdominal skin and fat with preservation of the rectus abdominus (or'sick-pack') muscle. This tissue is transferred to the chest to reconstruct the breast.

Current Herbs As Of Today

- Copper,po solid (copper gluconate), 2mg Capsule 1 PO QD
- Garlic, po solid, 400mg Tablet (s), enteric coated Take 1 PO daily.
- Iron, po solid, 18mg Tablet Take PO QD
- Selenium, po solid, 50 mcg Tablet Take 1 PO QD
- Turmeric (Curcumin), po solid, Capsule (s) Take 1 PO OD
- Vitamin B-12, po solid (cyanocobalamin) (vitamin b6)
- Zinc, po solid, 23 mg Lozenge (s) Take 1 PO QD

Type Of Treatment I Was On

First treatment: 10/10/2011 Last scheduled treatment day: 11/29/2011

Chemotherapy: Doxorubicin hcl, inj, Cyclophosphamide, inj &

Cyclophosphamide & Doxorubicin First treatment day: 12/12/2011 &

Last schedule treatment day: 01/09/2012

Capecitabine & Docetaxel: First treatment day: 01/17/2013 & Last

scheduled treatment day: 03/21/2013

My last day of Radiation was: 08/15/13

My healing journey has been a ride. I lost all of my body hair, and my teeth had become damage from the chemo, and the texture of my skin was very ugly to me when I looked into the mirror. The reflection staring back at me looked like a bloated fish starving for water. But today, my hair has grown back pretty, I have mini implants now with a beautiful smile, and waiting on the last surgery to complete my reconstruction. **"I'm Excited!"**

Dr. Teresa Graham's Personal Notes

Attention: My herbal regiments are not suggesting that you not follow your doctors order. I'm not promoting that they will cure your cancer, I'm just sharing what I did during my healing process. So, if God didn't tell you to throw those chemo pills away, please keep taking them.

Other Books By Dr. Teresa Graham

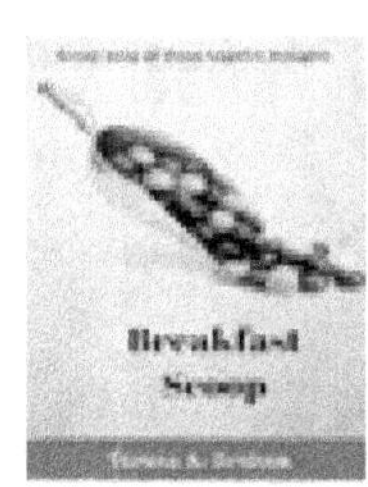
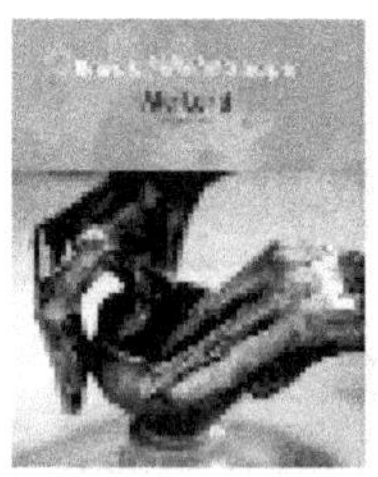

Breakfast Scoop & Break Mold Shape Me Lord: GET YOUR COPY TODAY!

NOTES

Chapter 1 - Where Do I Begin

King James Version

Chapter 2 - Shaken By Cancer

King James Version

National Academy of Science

Graeber, Thomas Ph.D.

Chapter 3 - Healing The Mind

King James Version

Dodie Osteen, Healed of Cancer

Chapter 4 - Why Did God Heal Boobs?

The National Cancer Institute

Dr. Teresa Graham's Personal Notes

Medline Plus

American Cancer Society

Chapter 5 - Cancer With A Vengeance

King James Version

Chapter 6 - Have Faith In God To Heal

King James Version

Chapter 7 - Take A Spiritual Dose Everyday

King James Version

Dr. Teresa Graham's Personal Notes

NOTES

NOTES

NOTES

breasts